POCKET ATLAS OF NORMAL CT ANATOMY OF THE HEAD AND BRAIN

Second Edition

Pocket Atlas of Normal CT Anatomy of the Head and Brain

Second Edition

Michelle M. Smith, MD

Associate Professor of Radiology and Otolaryngology
Chief of Head and Neck Neuroradiology
Department of Radiology
Medical College of Wisconsin and Froedtert Hospital
Milwaukee, Wisconsin

Timothy L. Smith, MD, MPH

Associate Professor of Otolaryngology
Chief of Rhinology and Laryngology
Department of Otolaryngology and Communication Sciences
Medical College of Wisconsin and Froedtert Hospital
Milwaukee, Wisconsin

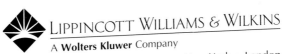

LIPPINCOTT WILLIAMS & WILKINS
A **Wolters Kluwer** Company
Philadelphia • Baltimore • New York • London
Buenos Aires • Hong Kong • Sydney • Tokyo

Acquisitions Editor: Joyce-Rachel John
Developmental Editor: Ellen DiFrancesco
Printer: Sheridan Press

© **2001 by LIPPINCOTT WILLIAMS & WILKINS**
530 Walnut Street
Philadelphia, PA 19106 USA
LWW.com

Printed in the USA

Library of Congress Cataloging-in-Publication Data
Smith, Michelle M.
  Pocket atlas of normal CT anatomy of the head and brain/Michelle M. Smith, Timothy L. Smith.—2nd ed.
    p. ; cm.
  Includes bibliographical references.
  ISBN-13: 978-0-7817-2949-9
  ISBN-10: 0-7817-2949-1
  1. Brain—Tomography—Atlases. 2. Head—Tomography—Atlases. I. Smith, Timothy L., MD. II. Title
  [DNLM: 1. Brain—anatomy & histology—Atlases. 2. Brain—anatomy & histology—Handbooks. 3. Brain—radiography—Atlases. 4. Brain—radiography— Handbooks. 5. Head—anatomy & histology—Atlases. 6. Head—anatomy & histology— Handbooks. 7. Head—radiography—Atlases. 8. Head—radiography—Handbooks. 9. Tomography, X-Ray Computed—Atlases. 10. Tomography, X-Ray Computed— Handbooks. WE 17 S655p 2000]
  QM455 .H337 2000
  611'.81'0222—dc21
                                                                    00-042122

10 9 8 7 6 5 4 3

Preface

Computed tomography (CT) has revolutionized cross-sectional imaging and has widespread applications in the head and neck and throughout the body.

Since the introduction of CT into clinical practice in the early 1970s, significant improvements in CT technology have been made. Modern conventional CT scanning can be performed at sub-millimeter collimation producing high-resolution images. More recently, with the introduction of spiral or helical CT, we are able to perform volumetric imaging. Reformatted images in the coronal and sagittal planes, and 3-D images can be generated from the axial data obtained with conventional or spiral CT. Multiplanar reformatted images can be particularly helpful in evaluation of the complex anatomy of the skull base, temporal bone, and sinonasal cavities of patients who cannot be positioned for direct coronal scanning.

This atlas demonstrates the normal anatomy seen in routine CT imaging of the brain, head, skull base, temporal bone, orbit, and sinonasal cavities. Prior to each individual section, the direction in which the scans proceed is indicated. Soft tissue and bone window images are included in the sections on the brain and calvarium, and orbit. Axial and coronal images are included in the temporal bone, orbit, and nasal cavity and paranasal sinus sections.

The atlas is intended for general radiologists, neuroradiologists, neurologists, neurosurgeons, otolaryngologists, and ophthalmologists. In particular, residents and fellows in training in these fields will find this book a useful reference. It is of utmost importance that specialists caring for patients with pathology of the brain and head understand the complex anatomy of this region.

Michelle M. Smith
Timothy L. Smith

Acknowledgements

The authors would like to thank the CT technologists at Medical College of Wisconsin–Froedtert Hospital and at the Center for Diagnostic Imaging in Milwaukee, WI for the time and effort they put into producing routinely high quality CT images. We would also like to thank the administrative assistants in the Department of Radiology and the Department of Otolaryngology and Communication Sciences at the Medical College of Wisconsin for their help in the preparation of this atlas.

Contents

Dedication

This atlas is dedicated to Bailey.

Brain and Calvarium

Images Proceed From Inferior to Superior

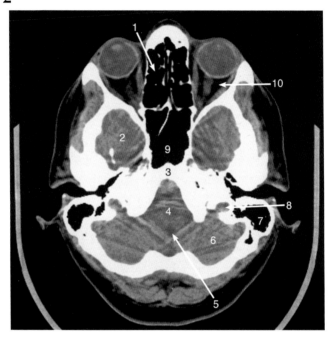

FIG. 1.
1. ethmoid air cells
2. temporal lobe
3. clivus
4. medulla
5. fourth ventricle
6. cerebellum
7. mastoid air cells
8. jugular foramen
9. sphenoid sinus
10. orbit

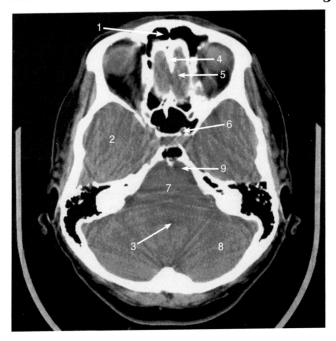

FIG. 2.
1. frontal sinus
2. temporal lobe
3. fourth ventricle
4. crista galli
5. gyrus rectus of frontal lobe
6. internal carotid artery
7. pons
8. cerebellum
9. prepontine cistern

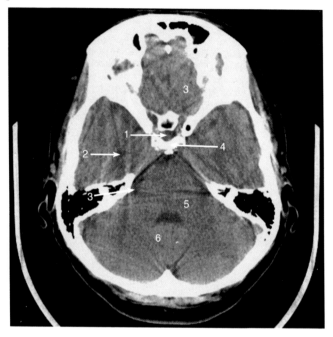

FIG. 3.
1. sella
2. temporal horn
3. frontal lobe
4. dorsum sella
5. middle cerebellar peduncle
6. cerebellar vermis
7. cerebello pontine angle cistern

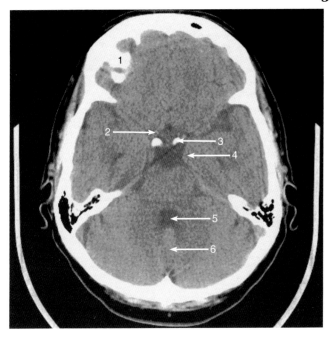

FIG. 4.
1. orbital roof
2. optic tract
3. posterior clinoid process
4. uncus of temporal lobe
5. fourth ventricle
6. cerebellar vermis

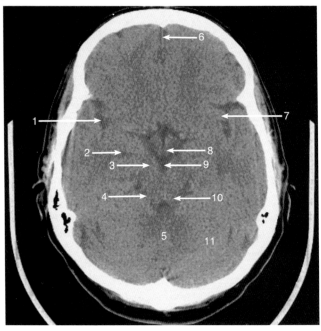

FIG. 5.
1. sylvian fissure
2. temporal horn
3. cerebral peduncle
4. ambient cistern
5. cerebellar vermis
6. falx cerebri
7. insula
8. mammillary body
9. interpeduncular fossa
10. midbrain tectum
11. cerebellar hemisphere

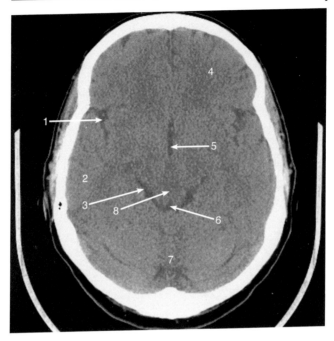

FIG. 6.
1. sylvian fissure
2. temporal lobe
3. ambient cistern
4. frontal lobe
5. third ventricle
6. quadrigeminal plate cistern
7. cerebellar vermis
8. midbrain

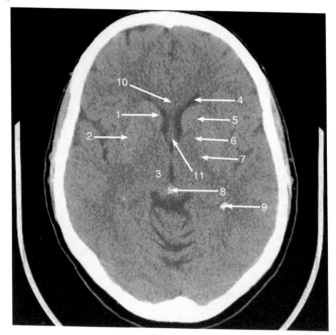

FIG. 7.
1. caudate head
2. putamen
3. thalamus
4. frontal horn of lateral ventricle
5. anterior limb of internal capsule
6. globus pallidus
7. posterior limb of internal capsule
8. calcified pineal gland
9. calcification in choroid plexus
10. genu of corpus callosum
11. foramen of Monro

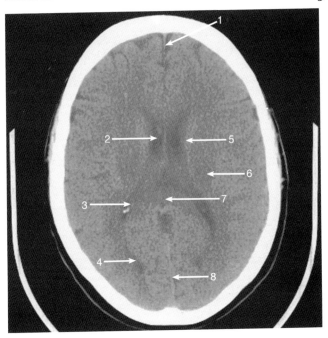

FIG. 8.
1. subarachnoid space
2. frontal horn of lateral ventricle
3. atrium of lateral ventricle
4. occipital horn of lateral ventricle
5. caudate body
6. corona radiata
7. splenium of corpus callosum
8. falx cerebri

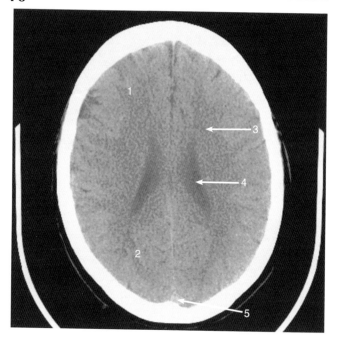

FIG. 9.
1. frontal lobe
2. parietal lobe
3. corona radiata
4. body of lateral ventricle
5. superior sagittal sinus

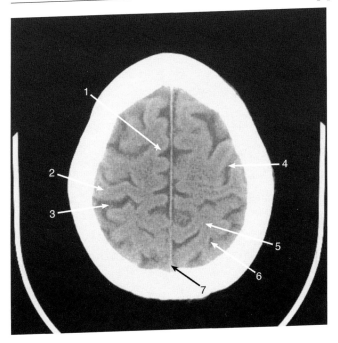

FIG. 10.
1. superior frontal gyrus
2. precentral gyrus
3. central sulcus
4. precentral sulcus
5. postcentral gyrus
6. intraparietal sulcus
7. superior sagittal sinus

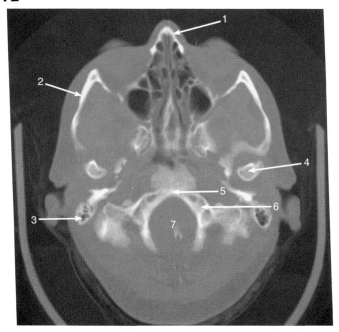

FIG. 11.
1. nasal bone
2. zygomatic arch
3. mastoid tip
4. mandibular condyle
5. clivus
6. hypoglossal canal
7. foramen magnum

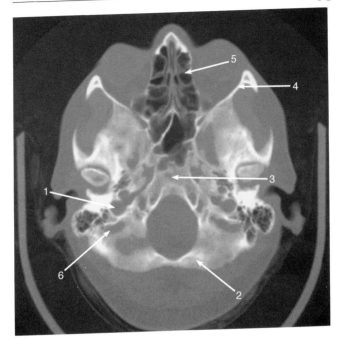

FIG. 12.
1. jugular foramen
2. occipital bone
3. clivus
4. lateral orbital wall
5. ethmoid sinus
6. groove for sigmoid sinus

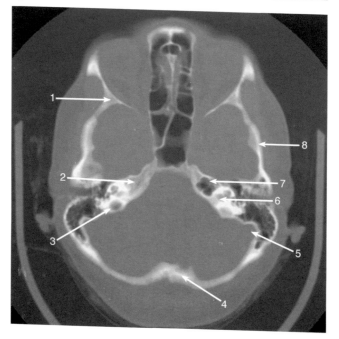

FIG. 13.
1. greater wing of sphenoid bone
2. petrous apex
3. cochlea
4. occipital bone
5. sigmoid groove
6. internal auditory canal
7. petrous apex air cells
8. squamous temporal bone

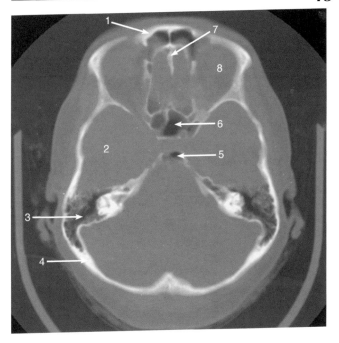

FIG. 14.
1. frontal bone
2. middle cranial fossa
3. mastoid cavity
4. occipitomastoid suture
5. dorsum sella (pneumatized)
6. sphenoid sinus
7. crista galli
8. orbit

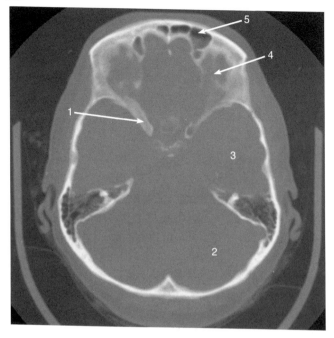

FIG. 15.
1. lesser wing of sphenoid bone
2. posterior cranial fossa
3. middle cranial fossa
4. orbital roof
5. frontal sinus

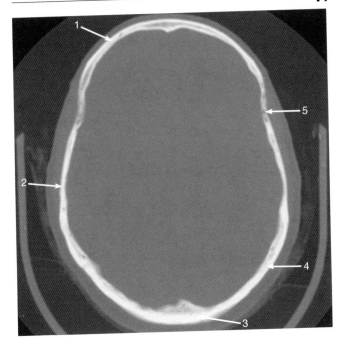

FIG. 16.
1. frontal bone
2. parietal bone
3. occipital bone
4. lambdoid suture
5. coronal suture

Brain and Calvarium

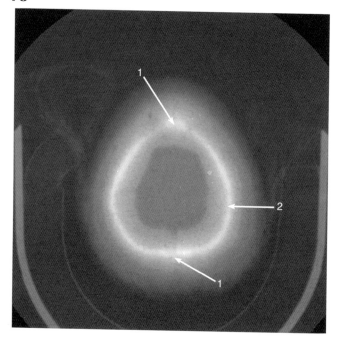

FIG. 17.
1. sagittal suture
2. parietal bone

Patient #

Name

DOB

Exam

Date/Time

Diagnosis

Doctor

Temporal Bone

Axial Images Proceed Inferior to Superior

Coronal Images Proceed Anterior to Posterior

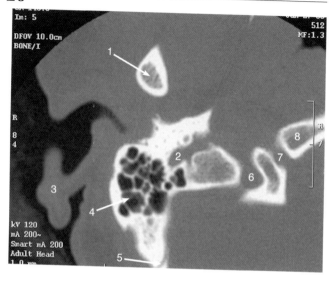

FIG. 18.
1. mandible (inferior aspect of condyle)
2. stylomastoid foramen
3. auricle
4. mastoid air cells
5. occipitomastoid suture
6. jugular foramen
7. hypoglossal canal
8. clivus

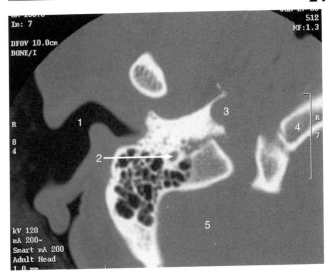

FIG. 19.
1. external acoustic meatus
2. mastoid (vertical) segment of facial nerve
3. jugular vein
4. clivus
5. posterior cranial fossa

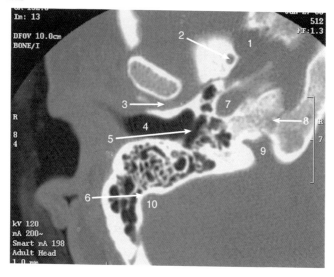

FIG. 20.
1. foramen ovale
2. foramen spinosum
3. temporomandibular joint
4. external auditory canal
5. tympanic membrane
6. sigmoid plate
7. carotid canal
8. petrooccipital synchondrosis
9. jugular foramen
10. sigmoid sinus

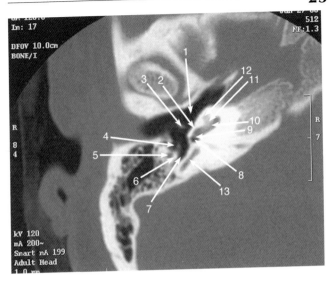

FIG. 21.
1. mesotympanum
2. cochlear promontory
3. manubrium of malleus
4. facial recess
5. facial nerve (mastoid segment)
6. pyramidal eminence
7. sinus tympani
8. round window niche
9. round window
10. basal turn of cochlea
11. middle turn of cochlea
12. apical turn of cochlea
13. posterior semicircular canal

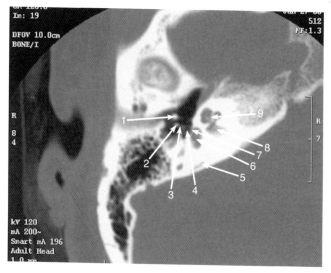

FIG. 22.
1. manubrium of malleus
2. lenticular process of incus
3. incudostapedial joint
4. crura of stapes
5. vestibular aqueduct
6. vestibule
7. oval window with stapes foot plate
8. internal auditory canal
9. cochlea

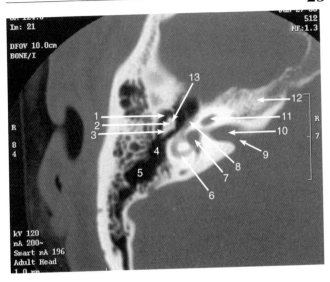

FIG. 23.
  1. epitympanum
  2. malleoincudal articulation
  3. body of incus
  4. aditus ad antrum
  5. mastoid antrum
  6. lateral semicircular canal
  7. vestibule
  8. tympanic segment of facial nerve
  9. porus acousticus
  10. internal auditory canal
  11. middle turn of cochlea
  12. petrous apex
  13. head of malleus

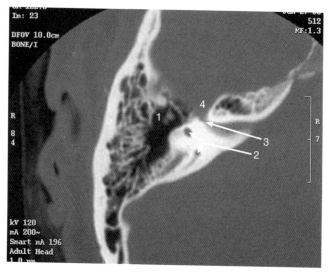

FIG. 24.
1. epitympanum
2. crura of superior semicircular canal
3. labyrinthine segment of facial nerve
4. geniculate ganglion

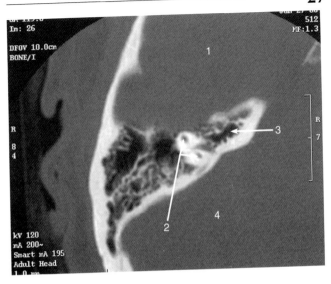

FIG. 25.
1. middle cranial fossa
2. superior semicircular canal
3. petrous apex air cells
4. posterior cranial fossa

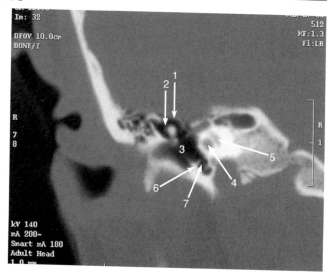

FIG. 26.
1. tegmen tympani
2. epitympanum
3. tympanic membrane
4. apical turn of cochlea
5. middle turn of cochlea
6. tympanic annulus
7. hypotympanum

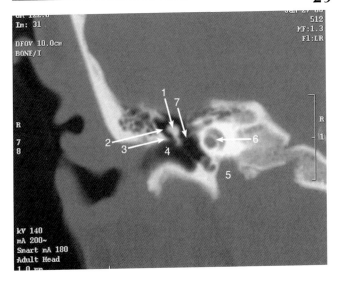

FIG. 27.
1. head of malleus
2. Prussak's space
3. scutum
4. external auditory canal
5. internal carotid artery
6. cochlea
7. tensor tympani tendon

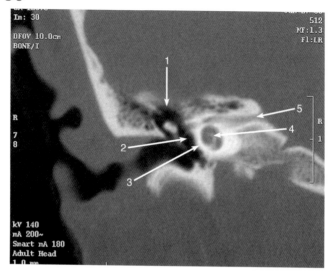

FIG. 28.
1. tegmen tympani
2. mesotympanum
3. cochlear promontory
4. cochlea
5. internal auditory canal

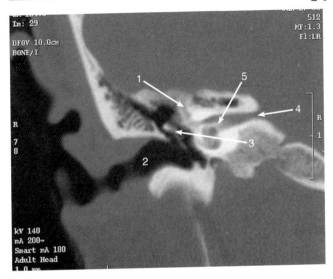

FIG. 29.
1. superior semicircular canal
2. external auditory canal
3. long process of incus
4. porus acousticus
5. crista falciformis

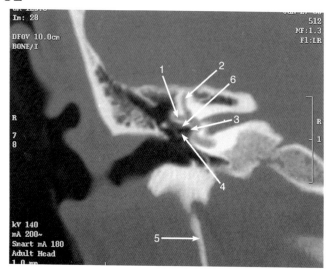

FIG. 30.
1. lateral semicircular canal
2. superior semicircular canal
3. oval window
4. stapes
5. styloid process
6. tympanic segment of facial nerve

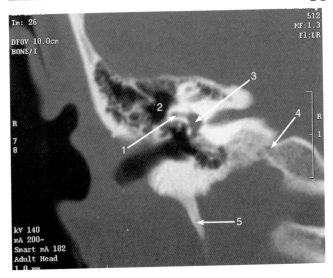

FIG. 31.
1. lateral semicircular canal
2. mastoid antrum
3. vestibule
4. petrooccipital synchondrosis
5. styloid process

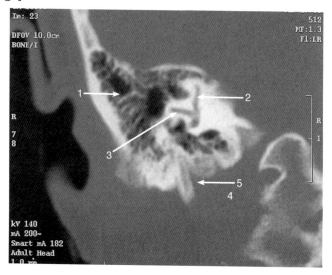

FIG. 32.
1. mastoid air cells
2. superior semicircular canal
3. lateral semicircular canal
4. jugular vein
5. stylomastoid foramen

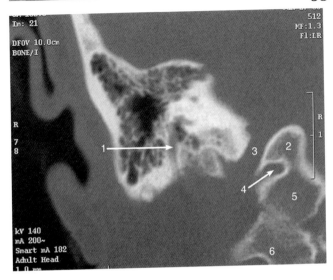

FIG. 33.
1. mastoid segment of facial nerve
2. jugular tubercle
3. jugular fossa
4. hypoglossal canal
5. occipital condyle
6. lateral mass of atlas (c1)

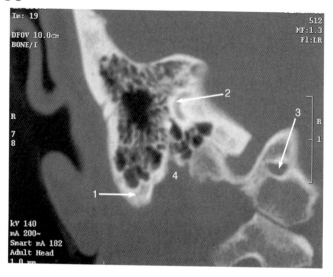

FIG. 34.
1. mastoid tip
2. posterior semicircular canal
3. hypoglossal canal
4. stylomastoid foramen

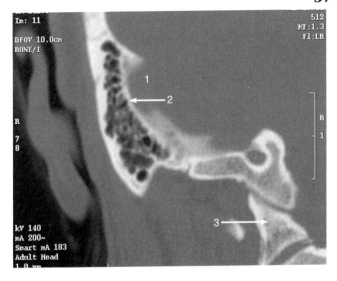

FIG. 35.
1. sigmoid sinus
2. sigmoid plate
3. lateral mass of atlas

Orbit

Axial Images Proceed From Superior to Inferior

Coronal Images Proceed from Anterior to Posterior

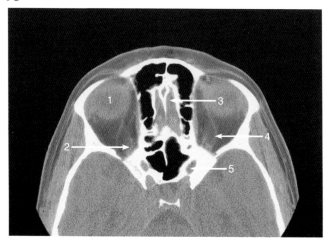

FIG. 36.
1. globe
2. posterior aspect of superior rectus muscle
3. gyrus rectus
4. superior ophthalmic vein
5. intracanalicular segment of optic nerve

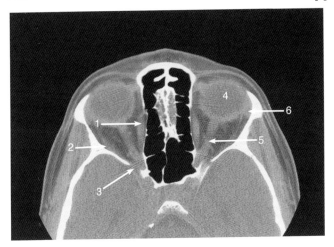

FIG. 37.
1. medial rectus muscle
2. lateral rectus muscle
3. superior orbital fissure
4. globe
5. optic nerve
6. lacrimal gland

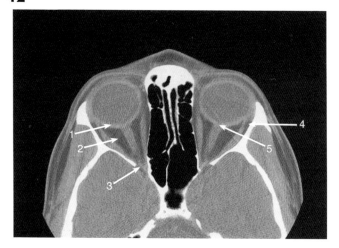

FIG. 38.
1. scleral layer of globe
2. intraconal fat
3. superior orbital fissure
4. extraconal fat
5. optic nerve insertion

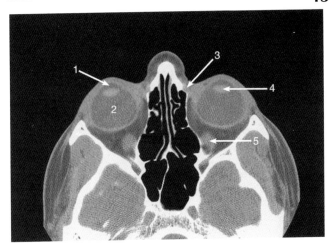

FIG. 39.
1. anterior chamber (aqueous body)
2. posterior chamber (vitreous body)
3. lacrimal sac
4. lens
5. inferior rectus muscle

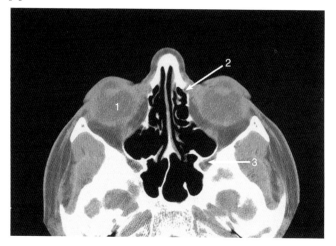

FIG. 40.
1. vitreous body
2. nasolacrimal duct (superior)
3. inferior orbital fissure

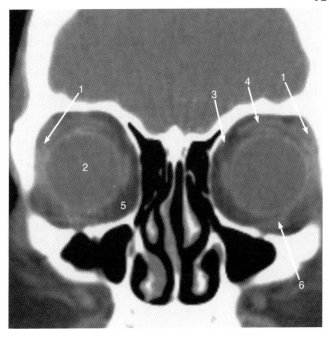

FIG. 41.
1. lacrimal gland
2. globe
3. superior oblique muscle
4. levator palpebrae muscle
5. intraorbital fat (extraconal)
6. inferior oblique muscle

Orbit

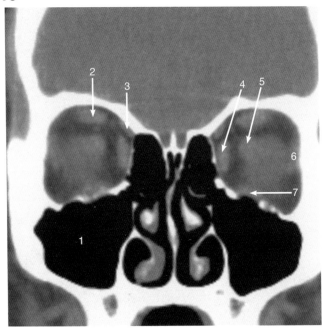

FIG. 42.
1. maxillary sinus
2. superior rectus muscle
3. superior oblique muscle
4. medial rectus muscle
5. optic nerve
6. lateral rectus muscle
7. inferior rectus muscle

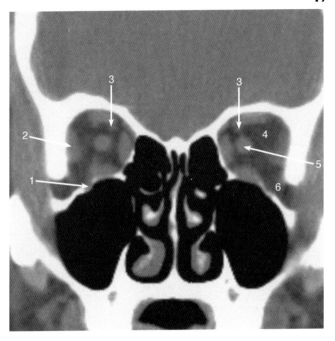

FIG. 43.
1. infraorbital nerve
2. lateral rectus muscle
3. superior ophthalmic vein
4. intraconal fat
5. optic nerve
6. inferior orbital fissure

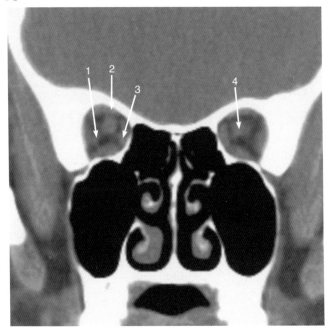

FIG. 44.
1. long posterior ciliary artery
2. superior rectus/levator palpebrae muscle complex
3. medial rectus muscle
4. optic nerve

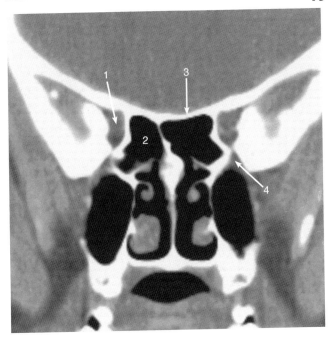

FIG. 45.
1. orbital apex
2. sphenoid sinus
3. planum sphenoidale
4. inferior orbital
   fissure

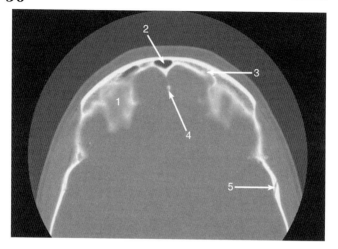

FIG. 46.
1. orbital roof
2. frontal sinus
3. frontal bone
4. crista galli
5. coronal suture

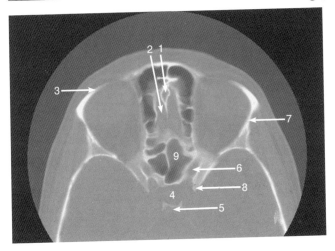

FIG. 47.
1. crista galli
2. gyrus rectus
3. superior orbital rim
4. sella
5. dorsum sella
6. optic canal
7. lateral orbital wall
8. anterior clinoid process
9. sphenoid sinus

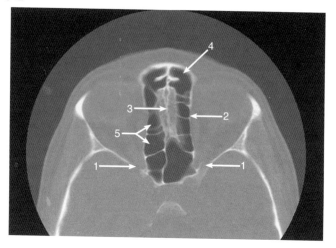

FIG. 48.
1. superior orbital fissure
2. lamina papyracea
3. perpendicular plate of ethmoid bone
4. frontal sinus
5. ethmoid air cells

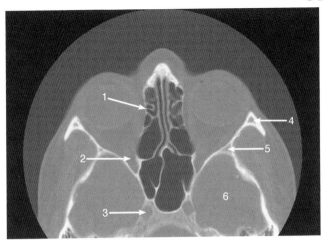

FIG. 49.
1. lamina papyracea
2. orbital apex
3. carotid canal
4. zygoma bone
5. greater wing of sphenoid bone
6. middle cranial fossa

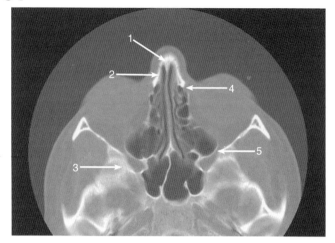

FIG. 50.
1. nasal bone
2. lacrimal bone
3. greater wing of sphenoid bone
4. lacrimal sac
5. inferior orbital fissure

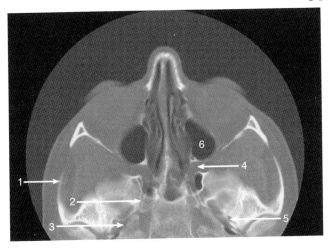

FIG. 51.
1. zygomatic arch
2. vidian canal
3. foramen lacerum
4. pterygopalatine fossa
5. foramen spinosum
6. maxillary sinus

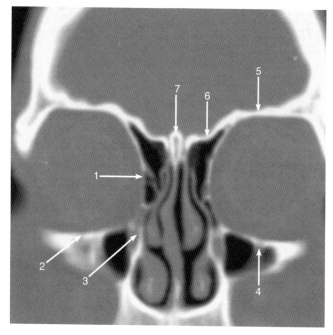

FIG. 52.
1. lamina papyracea
2. inferior orbital rim
3. nasolacrimal duct
4. infraorbital foramen
5. orbital roof
6. fovea ethmoidalis
7. crista galli

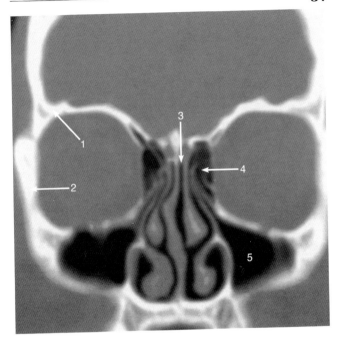

FIG. 53.

1. frontal bone
2. zygoma bone
3. cribriform plate
4. ethmoid labyrinth
5. maxillary sinus

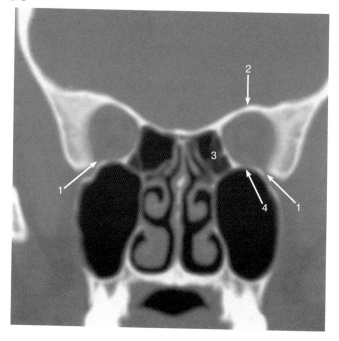

FIG. 54.
1. inferior orbital fissure
2. orbital roof
3. posterior ethmoid cells
4. maxillary bone

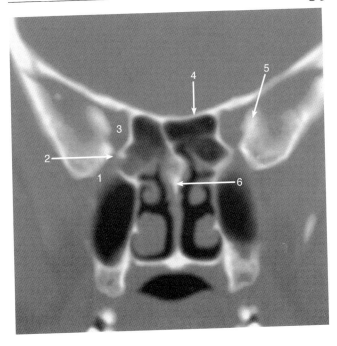

FIG. 55.
1. pterygomaxillary fissure
2. inferior orbital foramen
3. orbital apex
4. planum sphenoidale
5. greater wing of sphenoid bone
6. nasal septum

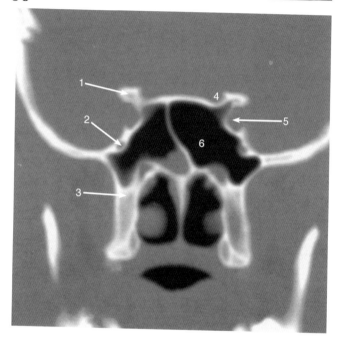

FIG. 56.
1. anterior clinoid process
2. foramen rotundum
3. pterygoid process
4. optic canal
5. superior orbital fissure
6. sphenoid sinus

Nasal Cavity and Paranasal Sinuses

Axial Images Proceed Inferior to Superior

Coronal Images Proceed Anterior to Posterior

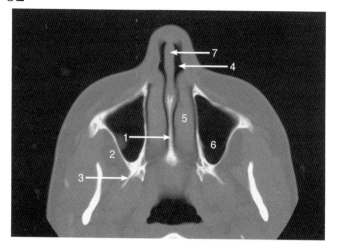

FIG. 57.
1. bony nasal septum
2. retroantral fat
3. lateral pterygoid plate
4. nasal vestibule
5. inferior turbinate
6. maxillary sinus antrum
7. cartilaginous nasal septum

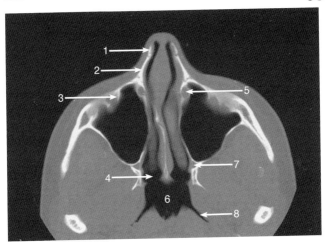

FIG. 58.
1. nasal bone
2. nasal process of maxilla
3. groove for infraorbital nerve
4. choanal opening
5. nasolacrimal duct
6. nasopharynx
7. sphenopalatine foramen
8. fossa of Rosenmüller

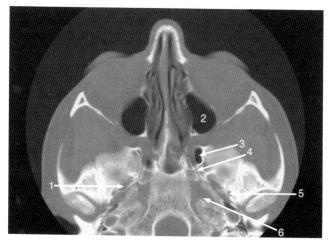

FIG. 59.
1. foramen ovale
2. maxillary sinus
3. pterygoid recess of sphenoid sinus
4. vidian (pterygoid) canal
5. foramen spinosum
6. foramen lacerum

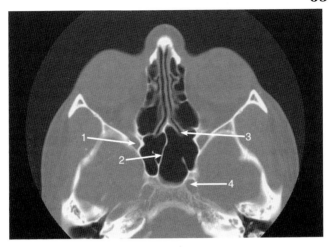

FIG. 60.
1. inferior orbital fissure
2. sphenoid septum
3. sphenoid ostium
4. internal carotid artery

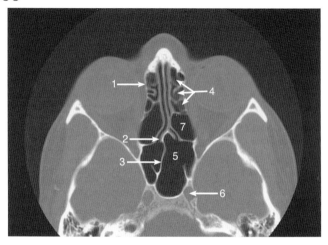

FIG. 61.
1. lamina papyracea
2. sphenoid ostium
3. sphenoid septum
4. anterior ethmoid air cells
5. sphenoid sinus
6. internal carotid artery
7. posterior ethmoid air cell

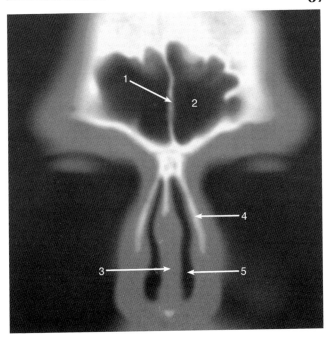

FIG. 62.
1. frontal sinus septum
2. frontal sinus
3. cartilagenous nasal septum
4. nasal bone
5. nasal vestibule

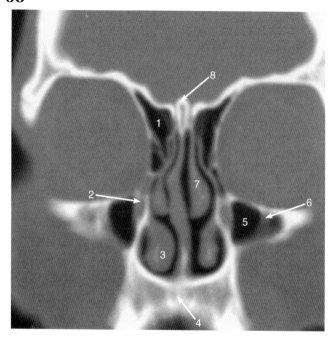

FIG. 63.
1. frontal sinus
2. nasolacrimal duct
3. inferior turbinate
4. hard palate
5. maxillary sinus
6. groove for infraorbital nerve
7. middle turbinate
8. crista galli

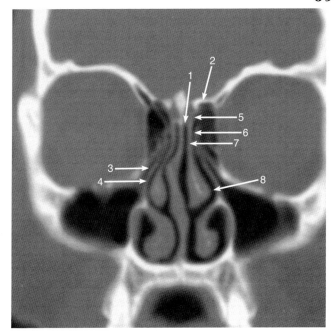

FIG. 64.
1. medial lamella of cribriform plate
2. fovea ethmoidalis
3. ethmoid infundibulum
4. uncinate process
5. lateral lamella of cribriform plate
6. frontal recess
7. vertical lamella of middle turbinate
8. middle meatus

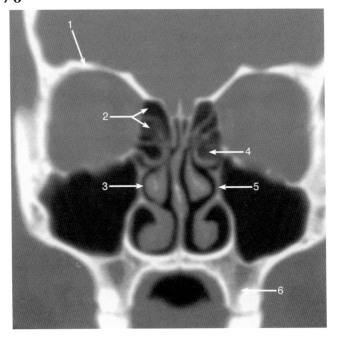

FIG. 65.
1. orbital roof
2. anterior ethmoid air cells
3. middle meatus
4. ethmoid bulla
5. uncinate process
6. superior alveolar ridge

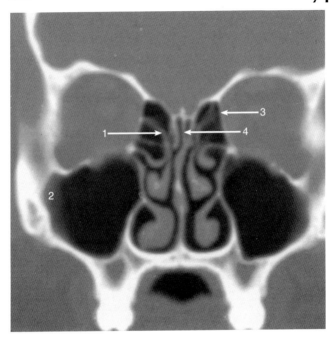

FIG. 66.
1. basal lamella (lateral lamella of middle turbinate)
2. lateral recess of maxillary sinus
3. lamina papyracea
4. perpendicular plate of ethmoid bone (superior nasal septum)

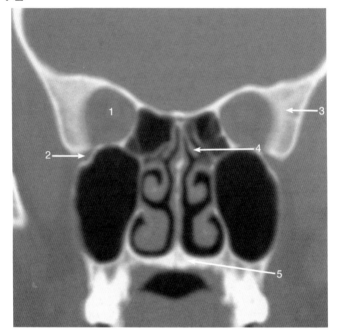

FIG. 67.
1. orbit
2. inferior orbital fissure
3. greater wing of sphenoid bone
4. superior turbinate
5. hard palate

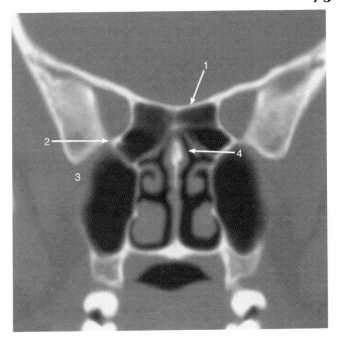

FIG. 68.
1. planum sphenoidale
2. inferior orbital fissure
3. infratemporal fossa
4. region of sphenoethmoidal recess

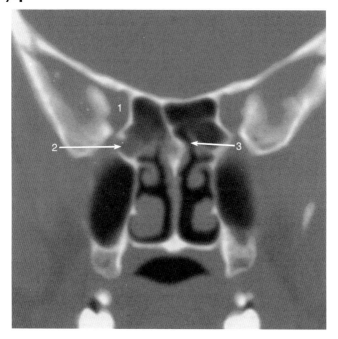

FIG. 69.
1. orbital apex
2. sphenopalatine foramen
3. sphenoid sinus ostium

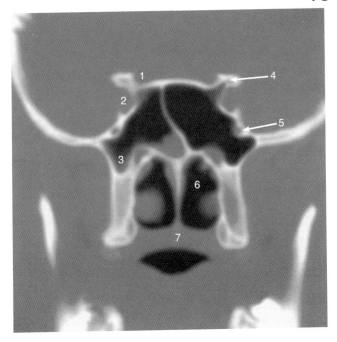

FIG. 70.
1. optic nerve
2. superior orbital fissure
3. pterygoid recess of sphenoid sinus
4. anterior clinoid process
5. foramen rotundum
6. choana
7. soft palate

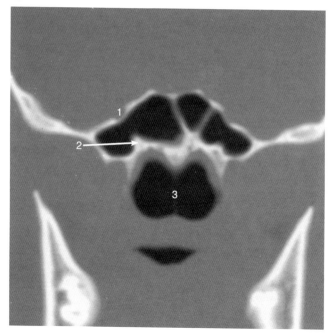

FIG. 71.
1. foramen rotundum
2. vidian canal
3. nasopharynx

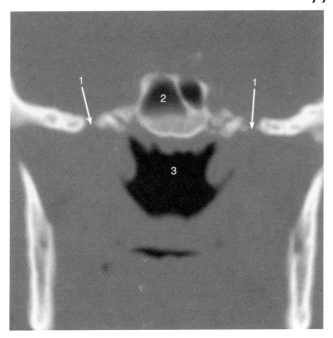

FIG. 72.
1. foramen ovale
2. sphenoid sinus
3. nasopharynx

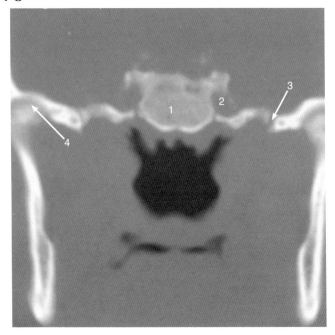

FIG. 73.
1. clivus
2. location of Meckel's cave
3. foramen spinosum
4. temporomandibular joint

References

1. Som PM, Curtin HD, eds. Head and Neck Imaging, 3rd ed. St. Louis: Mosby-Year Book, 1996.
2. Swartz JD, Harnsberger HR, eds. Imaging of the Temporal Bone, 2nd ed. New York: Thieme Medical Publishers, 1992.
3. Newton TH, Hasso AN, Dillon WP, eds. Modern Neuroradiology (Volume 3) Computed Tomography of the Head and Neck. Philadelphia: Raven Press, 1988.
4. Gentry LR, ed. Neuroimaging Clinics of North America: Normal Anatomy of the Brain, Head, and Neck. Philadelphia: W. B. Saunders, 1998.